Urine Testing for Marijuana Use: Implications for a Variety of Settings

AF676796

Edited by Margaret Blasinsky and George K. Russell, Ph.D.

Library of Congress Catalog Card Number: 82-198608
ISBN: 942348-02-8

Table of Contents

Introduction
by Robert L. DuPont, M.D. 5

I: Urine Testing for Marijuana Use–
Methods of Testing and Analysis 8

Marijuana–Factors in Testing 8
The EMIT Cannabinoid Assay Test 10
Radioimmunoassay for Cannabinoids 12

II: Summary of Technical Presentations and
Discussions 13

Introduction: Update on Marijuana
by Robert L. DuPont, M.D. 13
The Metabolism, Pharmacokinetics and Analysis
of Marijuana Components in Body Fluids:
Implications for Non-Research Use
by Richard Hawks, Ph.D. 15
Urinalysis Screening for Marijuana Use: Legal
and Ethical Considerations
by Nancy Wynstra 19
Implications for Public Policy: Ambivalence and
the Search for the "Magic Bullet"
by Richard H. Bucher, Ph.D. 24
Urine Testing for Marijuana: Implications for
Drug Treatment Programs
by Herbert Kleber, M.D. 26
Urine Testing for Marijuana Use, Implications in
Corrections
by Hugh Alcott 28

*Marijuana Testing–Implications for Highway
Safety* 31

Marijuana and Driving
by Herbert Moskowitz, Ph.D. 31
Marijuana and Highway Safety
by Arthur J. McBay, Ph.D. 32

Juvenile Marijuana Use 35
Remarks on Prevention
by William L. Barton 35
Urine Screen for Cannabinoids – A Pediatric View
by Donald I. Macdonald, M.D. 36
Implications of Urine Testing for Marijuana in a School Setting
by Richard A. Hawley, Ph.D. 37

Implications for Marijuana Testing in the Workplace and the Military 42
Urine Testing for Marijuana: Implications for the Workplace
by James L. Francek, MSW, ACSW 42
Remarks by Max P. Rogers, M.D. 44
Remarks by William C. Louisell, Brig. Gen., U.S. Army (Ret.) 45

Introduction

Robert L. DuPont, M.D.
President, American Council on Marijuana

Urine testing is the least glamorous and least developed but one of the most important aspects of drug abuse prevention. An understanding of the process of drug dependence is essential for understanding the potential of urine testing. A universal feature of the process which leads from curiosity and casual experimentation to full-blown drug dependence is *denial*. The drug user minimizes his use and the consequences of that use for himself and to others, particularly others who are likely to discourage his continued use of the drug. This is as true for the person who is dependent on alcohol or heroin as it is for the marijuana dependent person. Accordingly, there is a need for objective, clinical identification of marijuana use.

There are some features of marijuana use which set it apart from other drug dependencies. For example, in the United States over the last decade or two, cannabis has acquired a positive image, having become intertwined with the youth culture and with a false mythology which maintains that the drug is both harmless and not "addictive." In addition, marijuana, unlike virtually every other drug of abuse, has lacked an objective test for use. Urine testing for heroin, cocaine and other illegal drugs has played a central role in detection, treatment and prevention; the breath test for alcohol use, as well as blood and urine tests, have been vitally important in alcoholism treatment and prevention. But the lack of a simple test for marijuana use, coupled with societal ambivalence about the drug, has indirectly promoted widespread marijuana use.

During the last year, an inexpensive urine test has become available. The test was developed by the Syva Corporation and is now widely available in routine clinical laboratories throughout the United States. It is reliable and inexpensive. Collaborative Research, Inc. also supplies a urine testing kit, and others may be marketed in the future.

On December 12, 1980, the American Council on Marijuana held a one-day conference in Bethesda, Maryland to explore the implications of this new technology. The topics covered ranged from a review of the nature and extent of marijuana use to the technical, legal, and ethical issues in urine testing for marijuana use. The possible settings for the test ranged from drug prevention and treatment programs to prisons, and parole offices. Also considered were the role of parents, pediatricians, schools, and even highway patrols. While many questions were raised, and not all participants were equally enthusiastic about the new technology, there was broad agreement that the existence of this simple, effective test was indeed revolutionary. Careful consideration was urged with respect to technical issues (for example, making sure the specimen analyzed is actually from the subject being tested) and ethical issues (for example, consideration of privacy, due process, and informed consent) but the general conclusion was clear: this new technology deserves wide implementation.

One of the more interesting aspects of this new technology is that the urine test may be positive for marijuana constituents up to two weeks after a single use of the drug. This surprisingly long positive period is the result of the extended time the components of marijuana stay in the body after use of the drug. This can have a strong educational value for marijuana users: most are alarmed to learn that their bodies are being continuously exposed to these marijuana chemicals for weeks after the brief "high" is over. On the other hand the urine test does not distinguish between very recent use (e.g. use associated with the specific and short-lived "high") and use as distant as two weeks. While the test detects recent or current use it is not helpful in detecting acute intoxication. Prevention or treatment programs prefer this capability because urine need only be tested every two weeks to detect continuing use of the drug. This characteristic limits the test's usefulness in roadside or on-the-job testing, but this does not mean that the test is not useful in the latter settings. A negative test virtually rules out not only recent use but current intoxication. Roadside or on-the-job tests which produce a negative result show that the tested person is free of marijuana use. A positive test in such circumstances raises suspicion. (For confirmation of current intoxication, a blood test would be required, since blood levels correlate more directly with current intoxication).

The conference proceedings are summarized in this booklet, which, we believe, will prove useful to all who are considering using urine testing for marijuana use. Part I provides background information on the various methods for testing marijuana constituents and their metabolites in urine. Included is a discussion of the principal psychoactive ingredient in marijuana and how it is metabolized and eliminated from the body. Part II contains abstracts of the papers presented at the conference and highlights of related discussion topics.

Part I: Urine Testing for Marijuana Use – Methods of Testing and Analysis

There are at present two commercially available immunoassays for cannabinoid analysis in urine: the EMIT Cannabinboid Assay produced by Syva Company of Palo Alto, California and a radioimmunoassay (RIA) manufactured by Collaborative Research, Inc. of Waltham, Massachusetts.* Both are immunological methods, but the Syva assay detects cannabinoids by measuring enzyme activity with a spectrophotometer; the Collaborative Research method assays radioactivity with a scintillation counter. These assays are designed to detect metabolites found in urine resulting from the use of marijuana.

Analysis of cannabinoids can also be performed on blood samples. Methods for blood analysis include RIA and gas chromatography/mass spectrometry (GC/MS), which can also be used for analysis of urine.

While the conference panelists discussed the broad issues of testing for marijuana use, there was also specific focus on the new EMIT one-minute assay, designed for widespread use in urine testing.

MARIJUANA – FACTORS IN TESTING

Marijuana is a mixture of dried leaves and flowering tops of the plant *Cannabis sativa L.* The cannabinoid *delta-9-tetrahydrocannabinol* (delta-9-THC) is generally accepted to be the principal psychoactive ingredient in marijuana though other constituents may be important in modifying its effects, in addition to having their own physiological actions. The cannabis plant contains at least 61 different cannabinoids, and a total of 421 known chemicals.

"Street" preparations of marijuana tend to vary in

*Descriptive brochures are available from Syva Company, 900 Arastradero Road, P.O. Box 10058, Palo Alto, CA 94303 and Collaborative Research, Inc., 1365 Main Street, Waltham, MA 02154.

delta-9-THC content, the usual range being 0 to 5 percent. As marijuana has come to be more widely used, its detection in the human body has become an important chemical problem with major research and legal implications. Since many marijuana constituents are rapidly metabolized, and because of the very small quantities involved, the development of simple detection methods has been elusive.

Delta-9-THC is rapidly absorbed by inhalation and more slowly taken up from the gastrointestinal tract. It is almost completely metabolized. Less than one percent of this compound is recovered unchanged in the urine or feces, regardless of the route of administration. Accordingly, urine and feces primarily contain metabolites of THC. One of the prominent metabolites is 11-nor-delta-9-THC-9-carboxylic acid (9-carboxy-THC), which is present in plasma, feces, and urine, along with less well-defined metabolites. Most urinary constituents are acidic.

Studies with radioactive tracers have shown that over the first 72 hours, between 30% and 35% of metabolites are eliminated in the feces, the major route of excretion; and 10% to 15% are excreted in the urine. Therefore, even after 72 hours, 50% of the initial dose remains in the body. Much of the delta-9-THC which is not initially metabolized and excreted is probably distributed and absorbed by various fatty tissues, then slowly, after a much longer period of time, metabolized and excreted.

Smoking marijuana is the most effective route of administration. Psychoactive and physiological effects appear within minutes. The peak effect occurs in 20 to 30 minutes and the duration is about 90 to 120 minutes after smoking a single cigarette. The pharmacological effects are delayed when administration is by oral intake. Onset is usually 30 to 60 minutes after ingestion; peak effects occur in two to three hours; and the effects last three to five hours.

Blood levels of delta-9-THC peak in a few minutes after inhalation and within three hours after oral ingestion. These levels decline rapidly. Elevated excretion of urinary metabolites, however, occurs within hours after exposure to cannabinoids, and levels may remain detectable for three to 10 days after smoking. The major portion of metabolites is excreted within two days, though excretion continues slowly for more than one week. Delta-9-THC has been shown to be metabolized more rapidly in chronic users than in naive users, though no significant accumulation of drug or metabolites has been shown. It has been demonstrated, however, that frequent users often have basal values in their urine that exceed peak values obtained by relatively infrequent users.

The lack of correlation of psychoactive effects with urinary metabolite levels, together with variations in absorption and distribution of the drug, method of ingestion, and urinary volume, indicate that the assay of delta-9-THC metabolites in urine is useful only as an indicator of the recent use of cannabinoids and not as a measure of intoxication.

THE EMIT CANNABINOID ASSAY TEST

The EMIT Cannabinoid Assay is a rapid, semi-quantitative immunochemical test to detect the delta-9-THC by assay of its major urinary metabolites. The assay is designed as a rapid primary screening system, and a negative response is strong evidence that delta-9-THC metabolites are not present in excess of the detection limit (50 ng/ml)* of the assay. A positive test is strong evidence that delta-9-THC metabolites are present, thus indicating that the individual has recently smoked or ingested cannabis.

The EMIT Cannabinoid Assay Test is packaged in a kit containing sufficient chemicals to perform 100 tests, each test taking about one minute to perform. Thus, the EMIT test makes it possible to detect the presence of THC metabolites within minutes of receipt of the urine samples. Given its relative low cost (estimated at $175 per kit), and that urine samples can be analyzed in any office by trained personnel, without need to submit urines to a commercial or institutional laboratory, the EMIT process potentially has wide applicability for testing for marijuana use.

Technically, the EMIT Cannabinoid Assay is a homogeneous enzyme immunoassay designed to detect micro-amounts of THC metabolites in urine. A urine specimen is mixed with a reagent containing antibodies specific for cannabinoids; antibody binding occurs to any metabolite present. A second reagent containing an enzyme-labeled metabolite is introduced. When the enzyme-labeled drug binds to the antibody, catalytic activity of the enzyme on a substrate (also added) is reduced. Since amounts of antibody and enzyme-labeled metabolite are constant, the enzyme activity correlates with the concentration of metabolites in the sample. The reaction is measured with a spectrophotometer as an absorbance change resulting from the enzyme's catalytic action on the substrate.

*One nanogram (ng) is one billionth (10^{-9}) of a gram. Urinary concentrations are usually expressed as ng per milliliter (ml) of urine.

The assay is designed to detect 50 nanograms 11-nor-delta-9-THC-9-carboxylic acid (9-carboxy-THC) per ml of urine with greater than 95% confidence, as well as to detect urine containing no metabolites (0 ng/ml) as negative, with greater than 95% confidence.

Syva reports that the assay is "useful only as an indicator of recent use of cannabinoids and not as a measure of intoxication, since there are great variations in absorption and distribution of the drug, methods of ingestion, and urinary volume. It is also stated that "psychoactive effects do not correlate with urinary metabolite levels" and "positive results should be confirmed by an alternative method."

Syva has conducted several tests of the cannabinoid assay system. A study of eight selected populations identified 491 positive urine specimens from a total of 958 samples, indicating an overall positive urine incidence of 51% for these populations (taken from a methadone clinic, a prison, a parole center and a forensic toxicology lab).

In a second study, subjects were given two cigarettes, each containing 9 mg THC, which were smoked within a two-hour period. Cannabinoids were detectable in the urine four hours after initial drug use, and for up to 10 days following.

Syva also conducted controlled laboratory tests, in which drug-free urines were "spiked" with various levels of 9-carboxy-THC. Researchers reported that at least 95% of the samples containing the drug at or above the detection limit (50 ng/ml) gave a positive response, and at least 95% of the samples containing no drug gave a negative response.

In its summary report, Syva drew these conclusions:

> The precision of the EMIT Cannabinoid Assay is acceptable. Carry-over is not a problem in a well-maintained system, and the stability of the calibration curve over a working day is good.
>
> Accuracy was more difficult to assess, and was complicated by lack of an established and available reference method. Based on results from a smoking study and admission of use, accuracy is good. No false positives were observed in these situations. Analysis of spiked samples gave acceptable accuracy, although the conditions of sampling (pH of urine, time of collection, etc.) can affect semi-quantitation significantly.
>
> Specificity evaluation revealed no interference or significant cross-reactivity with a number of commonly encountered compounds.

Based on controlled smoking studies, detectable levels of cannabinoids are present in urine from four to 10 days after smoking. These data indicate that with the EMIT Cannabinoid Assay, it is not possible to distinguish very recent use (within 24 hours) from recent use (up to 10 days).

RADIOIMMUNOASSAY FOR CANNABINOIDS

A sensitive immunological method for the detection of delta-9-THC and other cannabinoids in urine samples has been developed by Collaborative Research, Inc. of Waltham, Massachusetts. This radioimmunoassay (RIA) is available as a complete kit, containing all of the necessary reagents. A liquid scintillation counter is used to determine radioactivity.

As stated by the company, "This RIA measures as little as 0.3 nanograms of the broad spectrum of cross reacting cannabinoids. Ideally suited to the detection of trace amounts in urine, the Collaborative Research system provides a simple method of large scale screening for THC abuse. The system is also applicable to chemotherapy associated nausea-suppression studies."

Other methods for detection of delta-9-THC and other cannabinoids are thoroughly reviewed in a N.I.D.A. publication entitled *Cannabinoid Assays in Humans.**

**Cannabinoid Assays in Humans*, National Institute on Drug Abuse Monograph 7 (1976), edited by Robert E. Willette, is available from NIDA, 11400 Rockville Pike, Rockville, Maryland 20852.

Part II: Summary of Technical Presentations and Discussions

This section provides abstracts of the papers presented during the ACM conference on the implications of urine testing for marijuana use. Also included are major discussion topics which elaborate on statements made in the formal presentations.

INTRODUCTION: UPDATE ON MARIJUANA

Robert L. DuPont, M.D.
President, American Council on Marijuana

In the context of the dramatic increase in marijuana, the increase in the potency of marijuana, and the increase in the scientific evidence on the health hazards of marijuana, what role can the new urine testing technology play in understanding and reducing the epidemic use of marijuana?

New technologies solve problems. They also create problems and provoke controversy. Too often we neglect to consider the implications of what we are doing, or review past experience in related areas. The new urine testing technology for marijuana use has potential in a variety of settings. But, as with any technology, it has limits as well as potential.

Today we want to explore the full range of these effects and summarize them in a useable fashion for potential users of this new test for recent marijuana use.

The following observations are significant for an understanding of the current drug picture in the United States.

- American young people are literally the only population in the history of the world in which large numbers of an entire generation have smoked marijuana.
- The health effects of smoking marijuana are weighed on a different scale from other health risks. Most new drugs are considered dangerous until proven safe. For marijuana, the assumption

has been the reverse.

- Marijuana is a far more powerful drug today than it was ten years ago when the average delta-9-THC potency was only one-half of one percent.
- When many of the early pronouncements about the harmlessness of marijuana were made, appropriate methodology had not yet been developed to study this extremely complex drug.

Statistics provided by the National Institute on Drug Abuse describe the current dimensions of the problem.

- In 1975, 5.7% of high school seniors were daily marijuana smokers and 5.7% were daily alcohol users (including beer). Five years later, the alcohol figure remained about the same, but daily marijuana use had almost doubled: One out of every eleven seniors were now smoking daily or almost daily – they averaged 3.5 "joints" per day, and 13% of these daily users smoked seven or more "joints" per day.
- Of the 49% of all seniors who smoked marijuana during the past year (1980), 39.8% said they usually stayed high three to six hours or more.
- Half of the marijuana smokers also used one or more other illegal drugs; among non-marijuana smokers, there were virtually no regular users of other illegal drugs.
- In the same five-year period, those seniors who admitted smoking by the ninth grade had increased from 17% to 31.4%.
- The data from the national survey of high school seniors may be "on the low side" because the survey does not include youngsters who do not reach their senior year nor youngsters who were not in school the day the survey was taken – students who may have become drop-outs or who were truant at the time, statuses which could be symptomatic of marijuana use.
- The 1979 national survey on drug abuse (ages 12 and older) showed that use of marijuana among 12- to 17-year-olds increased from 14% in 1971 to 30.9% in 1979. More than four million youngsters (16.7%) had smoked marijuana during the month prior to the survey, in contrast to 2.8 million in this age group who had smoked tobacco cigarettes. Among 16- and 17-year-olds, eight percent were daily or nearly daily users of marijuana.

- In 1962, only four percent of Americans ages 18 to 25 had ever used marijuana; by 1979, that figure was 68%, with more than one-third (35%) reporting use within the past month.
- In 1962, only two percent of Americans ages 25 to 36 had ever used marijuana; by 1979, that figure was 20%, with six percent reporting use in the previous month.
- There are four million youngsters 12 to 17 who are current users of marijuana; there are 11 million Americans 18 to 25 who use marijuana; and there are 8 million Americans 26 to 35 who use marijuana. This figure of 23 million current users is from 1979 data when the number of Americans who had ever used the drug at least once was 53 million.

Current marijuana statistics can be simply summarized:

- Marijuana use on a large scale has occurred only during the last two decades with most of the increase coming during the 1970's.
- Marijuana use begins as early as 12 years old with the most frequent ages of first use being 14 and 15. Use of the drug is less common over the age of 25 and is relatively infrequent over the age of 35.
- Today, in the United States, marijuana use by young people is comparable to levels of use of alcohol and tobacco and far exceeds the levels of use of any other illegal drug among members of this age group.

THE METABOLISM, PHARMACOKINETICS AND ANALYSIS OF MARIJUANA COMPONENTS IN BODY FLUIDS: IMPLICATION FOR NON-RESEARCH USE

Richard Hawks, Ph.D.
Division of Research, National Institute on Drug Abuse (NIDA)

Metabolic Facts

Easy detection of marijuana use or intoxication would facilitate drug treatment counseling and provide a broader data base by which to assess marijuana's impact on health, and traffic and industrial safety. It has been difficult to develop methods suitable for the routine detection of marijuana use among groups which are considered to be in a relatively high risk situation either to themselves or society.

NIDA has been actively pursuing the development of such methods to facilitate basic research programs on marijuana toxicity, pharmacokinetics and studies on the extent of marijuana's impact on driving safety. In order to understand the uses and limitations of methods for the analysis of marijuana components in body fluids, it is necessary to know something about the metabolism and pharmacokinetics of the plant's primary psychoactive component, delta-9-tetrahydrocannabinol (delta-9-THC).

When marijuana is smoked, about 30% of the THC in the cigarette is taken into the lungs. A portion of this rapidly enters the blood stream, creating the "high" which starts within minutes of smoking and lasts for about one to two hours. THC is carried by the blood through the liver where some of it is transformed enzymatically to several metabolites. Most of these metabolites then enter body systems for eventual elimination by fecal or urinary routes. A typical graph of blood concentration versus time shows that the THC reaches high levels rapidly and decreases to about half of its concentration every 45–70 minutes. This latter measure is known as the "half-life" of THC in the blood.

The metabolite found in highest concentration in blood is 11-nor-delta-9-THC-carboxylic acid (9-carboxy-THC). This metabolite persists in the blood for a much longer time than THC itself.

Experiments using radioactive THC administered intravenously indicate that 50% of the dose is excreted in urine and feces in approximately three days. The remainder of the dose is thought to be absorbed by various fatty tissues of the body and then gradually excreted.

Almost no THC appears in the urine as unchanged parent drug. The major metabolites are acid derivatives and predominant among these, as in blood, is 9-carboxy-THC. Detection of acid metabolites in urine is possible even when blood levels drop below the limit of assay sensitivity, because of the concentrating action of the kidneys.

In blood, both THC and its longer persisting metabolite, 9-carboxy-THC, can be measured by several different analytical methods. Since THC enters the blood stream rapidly from the lung and disappears in a few hours, the determination of intoxication by blood concentration is a possibility. However, because of individual variability and tolerance phenomena, it may be impossible to cite a specific blood concentration of delta-9-THC above which most individuals could be presumed to be impaired.

In urine, THC is generally undetectable and primary manifestations of the parent drug are the various acid metabolites, including 9-carboxy-THC. The information derived from a urine assay of THC metabolites concerns the incidence of drug use. Since the metabolites enter the urinary excretion system one to two hours after ingestion and persist for several days, a positive urine analysis indicates that marijuana has been used, but, regardless of the actual amounts of metabolites measured, the time of ingestion cannot be fixed more precisely than from one hour to several days prior to the time of assay. This obviously precludes any determination of intoxication from a urine test.

Assay Methods

Several radioimmunological methods have been developed which are highly specific for THC or 9-carboxy-THC. Equally sensitive and specific is gas chromatography/mass spectrometry. It is much more expensive, however. EMIT methodology is relatively inexpensive but is currently limited to urine.

The EMIT system is, at the present time, the most convenient commercial assay available for the detection of cannabinoid metabolites in urine. The method is convenient because it can be performed quickly (one minute) on a small (50 microliter) urine sample. This method is an immunologically-based procedure which provides a measure of the competition for a specific antibody "receptor" site between cannabinoid metabolites in a urine sample and a measurable chemical competitor for those sites.

The sensitivity of an assay is a measure of the least amount of material the assay will reliably detect. This has been determined in the case of the EMIT assay by assaying 50 urine samples free of cannabinoids before and after they are spiked with a known quantity of 9-carboxy-THC. Syva has determined that a 50 ng/ml concentration is the level of drug which provides a 95% confidence that the instrument readout will exceed that of any of the 50 blank samples.

The specificity of an assay is a measure of its ability to distinguish the target drug from other drugs which might appear in the samples. In the case of the EMIT assay, the target is a group of cannabinoid metabolites related in structure to 9-carboxy-THC. Test samples containing known amounts of many other common drugs have been tested and the EMIT system shown to be unresponsive to them.

In an attempt to assess better the reliability of this method, NIDA carried out an evaluation project involving 12 forensic laboratories which agreed to screen urine samples. The EMIT system has proven to be reliable within specified sensitivity limits and in the analysis of field samples from this evaluation study.

Conclusion

In order to prove true reliability in routine laboratory testing, many more "real" samples need to be analyzed and confirmed by alternate methods such as GC/MS. The reliability is at present, however, quite sufficient for research purposes. The use of the method as a forensic tool must be somewhat qualified, however. Regardless of the tested reliability of the system and the experience of the technician operator, false positive results are always a possibility with any assay. The possibility of such an event with the EMIT system appears to be quite low but insufficient data are available to say exactly what it is.

The inherent possibility of error in any assay is a matter of concern which escalates in proportion to the consequences of the positive result. A false positive result occurring once in 100 true positives is insignificant in an incidence survey for research purposes. The one false positive is of grave concern, however, if it is a forensic sample from an individual whose freedom, career or civil rights hang in the balance.

In forensic science, such occurrences are minimized to levels of little concern by the use of confirmatory methods of analysis. High confidence can be placed on a urine sample which is drug positive by an immunoassay method, such as EMIT, if it is also positive by a method based on completely different principles, such as GC/MS.

For all practical purposes, there is not, at present, a simple confirmatory assay generally available for the positive urinalysis. This fact seems to draw an obvious line in terms of the limitations on where EMIT can be used and where its use becomes scientifically and ethically questionable.

If the consequences of a positive EMIT analysis will impinge significantly on the individual, its use in the absence of corroborating data is inappropriate. Otherwise, as a counseling tool, a research tool, or a diagnostic tool, EMIT could be quite useful and appropriate where incidence of use and not intoxication is the question.

Finally, the perspective of how marijuana fits into general substance abuse must not be lost. Studies designed to screen for alcohol, marijuana, and other drugs in injured and erratic drivers have consistently shown that in the portion of cases where marijuana components are detected, alcohol and/or other drugs are usually also present.

It has also been reported that an individual's urine level of cannabinoid metabolites as analyzed by EMIT may remain significantly high for greater than two weeks. These levels can also fluctuate greatly due to fluctuations in urine volume at any given time. In a study of six subjects who had ingested two marijuana cigarettes, EMIT analysis of twice daily urine samples showed fluctuations from negative values (at 20 ng cut-off) to as high as 75–100 ng/ml one or two days later. In two subjects, urine samples separated by five days were assayed for higher values at the later time. These types of fluctuations have to be considered whenever periodic monitoring is carried out over days (or even weeks in the case of a formerly heavy chronic smoker). Increases in urine concentrations indicated by samples taken a week apart do not necessarily prove that the individual has taken marijuana during that time.

URINALYSIS SCREENING FOR MARIJUANA USE: LEGAL AND ETHICAL CONSIDERATIONS

Nancy Wynstra
General Counsel, Michael Reese Hospital and Medical Center, Chicago, Illinois

There are few easy answers to the question of whether urine testing for marijuana use is legal. The drug-crime connection, real or perceived, which provided much of the rationale for widespread testing for opiates and other illicit drugs in the urine of arrestees, probationers or parolees, seems to be absent when the drug of abuse is marijuana. One factor which will impact on the ethical, if not the legal, issues involved in deciding on how to use this new technique is that marijuana use is, apparently, far more prevalent than the use of any other "illicit" drug, and its use is widely accepted, as evidenced by the fact that marijuana possession for personal use has been decriminalized in at least 12 states. It would be incongruous indeed to embark on an elaborate screening program to identify marijuana users in those states where the only penalty for such use is a civil fine. Even in those states where marijuana possession is a misdemeanor, it seems unlikely that mandatory testing of the general population or of all arrestees to obtain evidence for criminal prosecution would withstand legal challenge, or that such a program would be desirable even if legally supportable.

Most people, even those who disapprove of its use,

do not seem to view severe criminal sanctions as the appropriate way to deal with marijuana use. Such use is often equated with alcohol use and, even where marijuana remains illegal, the use is tolerated, and often socially accepted or even encouraged. To the extent marijuana has a negative image, it is more generally associated (like alcohol) with offensive behavior and traffic accidents than with "serious" crime. Thus, it is difficult to imagine the public accepting a program which would screen the general population for the use of alcohol or pot.

Now that a test is available to identify the presence of marijuana metabolites in the urine, it is important to consider the legal implications of this new technology. In assessing potential legal problems, it is clear that the legality of urine testing for marijuana use will vary depending on the extent and circumstances of the testing and the use made of information collected.

Thus, to determine the probable legality of any specific marijuana testing program, several aspects of the program must be analyzed. The questions to be asked include:

(1) Who is being tested?

Possible groups to be tested include: the general population; persons arrested for a variety of crimes, including where applicable, public inebriation, or disorderly conduct; persons charged with various traffic offenses including driving while intoxicated; probationers and parolees; school children; employees; athletes; or virtually any other subgroup. The more broad the net of testing extends, the more difficult it will be to support the legality of the program.

(2) Who is doing the testing?

Testing could be done by law enforcement officials; public health officials; regulatory agencies; or others. The extent to which testing is done by qualified individuals and under appropriate conditions will impact on the legality of any testing program.

(3) Why is the testing being done?

Testing may be done to identify marijuana users for subsequent criminal or civil enforcement action; to identify candidates for treatment; to screen job applicants; to assess blame in vehicular accidents; to reduce accidents; or simply to obtain information on the extent of marijuana use. Test to support criminal action is probably suspect and testing to identify users, with no follow-up, raises ethical problems. Testing to refer to treatment is valid only if treatment is available and efficacious.

(4) How are the test results used?
Mandatory tests which form the basis for a subsequent criminal prosecution appear unlikely to withstand constitutional challenge while voluntary tests used for statistical purposes or to screen entrance into treatment programs are probably acceptable. Use of test results for pre-employment screening or to determine eligibility for sports competition or advancement in military rank pose other possible legal problems and could be challenged on equal protection or other grounds. Public dissemination of test results appears to violate not only federal confidentiality requirements, but legitimate privacy expectations.

The applicability of several legal principles must be assessed to determine whether any particular testing program would be likely to withstand legal challenge. The core issues are the following:

1. Privacy

Although the Constitution does not explicitly mention any right of privacy, the protections of the Constitution have been held to extend to certain areas or "penumbras" of privacy. Wrongful intrusion into one's personal affairs and private activities constitute an invasion of privacy. It is only when the individual's conduct begins to affect a third party or society at large that intervention into the "zone of privacy" becomes warranted.

It could be argued that a widespread testing program for a drug as extensively used as marijuana inappropriately invades an individual's zone of privacy. Despite the legitimate government interest in identifying drug users in the general population, it is unlikely that this interest, which is surely no greater than the interest in identifying people who have committed other crimes, would be regarded as sufficiently strong to support mass screening of groups of people who are suspected of no other crime. The general interest in deterring crime has never been regarded as sufficient to overcome the Fourth Amendment's limitations on the pursuit of criminals to methods which are not grossly intrusive into an individual's privacy.

2. Due Process

The due process clause of the Fourteenth Amendment requires that persons not be deprived of life, liberty or property without due process of law. In order for a testing procedure to withstand a due process challenge, it would be necessary that the tests be conducted in accordance with sound medical procedures and that the degree of bodily invasion be as minimal as possible under the circumstances. Although there are no known cases dealing specifically with the question of compelled urinalysis (except under the implied consent provisions of state traffic laws), the Supreme Court has upheld taking blood specimens from unconscious and unconsenting drivers.

Based on (Rochin v. California) standards, it is unlikely that requiring arrested individuals to provide voluntarily expelled urine specimens would violate the due process clause.

3. Self Incrimination

The Fifth Amendment generally protects a person from being forced to incriminate himself. While urine testing may produce information which could be the basis for a criminal prosecution, the courts have generally limited the protection against self-incrimination to testimonial evidence and have held that physical evidence, including body fluids, is not protected under the Fifth Amendment.

The key case in this area is Schmerber v. California. On this basis it seems unlikely that a testing program would be struck down on Fifth Amendment grounds, although some state courts refuse to allow as evidence the fact that a defendant has refused to submit to chemical testing.

4. Search and Seizure

The Fourth Amendment protects "the right of the people to be secure in their persons, houses, papers, and effects, against unreasonable searches and seizures." Although no courts appear to have considered the issue, it seems likely that the collection of urine specimens would be regarded as a search or seizure.

To withstand Fourth Amendment challenges it is necessary that the search or seizure be reasonable, and with a few exceptions, any search conducted without a judicial warrant is deemed unreasonable. Clearly, a requirement of obtaining a judicial warrant before each test would make any broad scale urine screening program administratively unworkable. Moreover, no showing of probable cause would be made to support the issuance of a warrant if the defendant showed no symptoms of drug use.

Thus, it is necessary to determine whether such a program might fall within one of the exceptions to the warrant requirement: (a) investigatory searches; (b) searches incident to arrest; and (c) administrative searches.

5. Implied Consent

It is generally agreed that a person may waive any constitutional right and that illegal searches are cured by the voluntary consent of the one being searched. To deal with problems of drunk driving, all states have enacted statutes providing that any person who operates a motor vehicle upon the public highways is deemed to have consented to a chemical test of his blood, breath, urine or saliva, to determine the alcoholic content, whenever he is arrested for an offense involving a motor vehicle while intoxicated and the arresting officer has reasonable grounds to believe that the person was driving while under the influence of alcohol.

The probative value of evidence indicating intoxication is directly related to the passage of time between the alleged offense and the administration of the test, so that the test must be administered near the time of the offense. The rationale supporting this time requirement (in Illinois statutes) is that the effects of alcohol ingestion upon motor coordination have a limited duration. The fact that a person was inebriated three days prior to or three days after the alleged offense is irrelevant.

This time sequence is one problem with the proposed EMIT assay. Clinical Study No. 74 indicates: "Based on controlled smoking studies, detectable levels of cannabinoids are present in urine from four to ten days after smoking." These data indicate that with the EMIT Cannabinoid Assay it is not possible to distinguish very recent use (within 24 hours) from recent use (up to 10 days).

No writer on the subject has theorized that motor coordination impairment stemming from marijuana ingestion can last 10 days. In fact, several hours is the generally accepted time period. Therefore, in regards to traffic violator submission to the proposed urine test, any evidence obtained would have no probative value. However, assuming a test was devised to measure marijuana ingestion within a relevant time period, any constitutional challenge could be overcome.

Provided that necessary safeguards are written into the proposal, a law calling for blood or urine analysis of one lawfully arrested for driving under the influence of marijuana should overcome a Fourth Amendment unreasonable search and seizure challenge.

Conclusion

It is clear from the preceding summary analysis of the legal implications of urine testing for marijuana use that there are no uniform answers. The legality will be determined on the basis of who is being tested, under what circumstances, and with what results. The likelihood of withstanding a legal challenge will be greatest if the test program is narrowly drawn and its focus rehabilitative rather than punitive, although it may not be meaningful to talk of addiction or rehabilitation in the context of marijuana use.

Any testing program will be evaluated on its individual merits with the court looking, ultimately, at the reasonableness of the balance struck between, on the one hand, the right to individual privacy and each individual citizen's right to be left alone, and on the other hand, the need to deal with the perceived problem of marijuana use in various populations.

IMPLICATIONS FOR PUBLIC POLICY: AMBIVALENCE AND THE SEARCH FOR THE "MAGIC BULLET"

Richard H. Bucher, Ph.D.

The only consistent societal message regarding the use of substances such as alcohol, cigarettes, opium, marijuana and other "recreational" drugs has concerned the use by children and adolescents. By and large the U.S. society is willing to impose, and occasionally enforce, sanctions and controls to limit psychoactive drug use by youth. For example, all states and most municipalities prohibit the sale of alcohol and tobacco products to minors. Many communities and states prohibit the use of drugs by minors and can impose civil and criminal penalties on adults when minors are found to be using the substance in a home when an adult is present, or in a bar or a restaurant which serves alcohol.

One point is abundantly clear: Americans use psychoactive substances on a large scale. General prevalence figures for drug, alcohol and tobacco use within society reflect, at best, a modest success for the general sanction efforts of society. Yet, society seems reluctant to impose more direct controls.

There have been few attempts to effect social controls designed to identify specific individuals whose only targeted behavior is the use of psychoactive substances. Usually such attempts are aimed at people who are also involved in other antisocial behavior. One could make a strong argument that society has been unwilling to cross the threshhold of control except in very circumscribed instances, usually involving after-the-fact controls (e.g., driving under the influence, disorderly conduct, etc.).

Any drug use is the result of partially understood and clearly complex sets of behaviors, attitudes and relationships. Marijuana use is no different. The question at hand is: What do we hope to achieve by identifying marijuana users? There are several observations which can be made regarding the public policy implications of control mechanisms. It appears there have evolved two criteria for the imposition of control. First, there must be a substantial and clear threat to a vulnerable part of society, the threat being of such a nature as to weaken substantially the value society places on that segment. Second, when approval is given, it is for limited application of the sanctions.

In all cases where control mechanisms have involved urinalysis, there has been controversy and opposition to the desirability of specific control, especially the use of urinalysis.

Even when there are substantial data that suggest that urinalysis does act as an effective deterrent to drug use, the price of that technique is often deemed too high by society. This opinion appears to be shared by policymakers.

This reluctance indicates a resistance to apply clearly established techniques which will identify people engaging in specific socially undesirable behavior, but without other consequence.

While acknowledging the negative social consequences of drug use, society does not appear to be ready to apply extraordinary measures to reduce it; underlying values of privacy and individual liberties dominate considerations of control. There may be legal precedent for this action, but no one is rushing to use it. In my view, this social reluctance reflects an implicit recognition by society that there is no "magic bullet" and that current social and medical responses to drug abuse are only marginally successful.

If this is the case, then the question should be asked if we want to encourage a technique of social control when we may not be able constructively to help those identified. For example, if only 20% of those 18–25 year olds currently (within the last 30 days) using cannabis in the armed services were identified, over 50,000 more people would be referred to military drug abuse programs. Or, if only 20% of high school seniors currently smoking marijuana (within the last 30 days) were identified, over 200,000 youth would be available for referral to school or other community services.

What would be the nature of these responses? Are we confident that the good which could come from such referrals will outweigh the negative consequences in terms of social stigma and arbitrary and capricious responses? We could ask similar questions regarding testing within the workforce and elsewhere.

It seems that while society may wish to lessen the impact of drug use, especially marijuana use, it does not have reasonable non-punitive programs available which clearly work and which have the confidence of the community. Identification may be a first good step in addressing the problem, but if little of substance follows identification, the response may well take on a futile meaning and contribute to the social confusion surrounding the problem.

Consequently, it seems to me that cannabinoid testing is an issue which can gain public support only if it is applied to that segment of the population which is truly vulnerable, and then only if the social or political threat is deemed to be substantial or subverting to health, morals or security of the nation. Segments of the military, others in a position of trust and authority (police, firemen) and those with a direct responsibility for the lives of others (pilots, railroad engineers, bus drivers, etc.) seem to constitute vulnerable groups.

The issue of testing in the workplace will be decided around questions of job security. In all other areas, the public concern for individual liberties will likely prevail since the precedents created by widespread cannabinoid testing in schools, on the highways or elsewhere could cut directly against the generally accepted rules of social conduct.

URINE TESTING FOR MARIJUANA: IMPLICATIONS FOR DRUG TREATMENT PROGRAMS

Herbert Kleber, M.D.,
Professor of Psychiatry, Yale Medical School,
and Director, Substance Abuse Treatment Unit,
Connecticut Mental Health Center

The impact of the new urine test for marijuana will be quite varied. For some treatment programs, the effects will be minimal and the test scarcely used; for others, it will be a useful treatment adjunct; and for some others, the negative impact may outweigh any positive value.

Methadone maintenance programs usually take the position that marijuana, while not desirable, is a lesser evil and make no great effort to combat its use. Therapeutic communities often deal with the polydrug user as well as the heroin abuser, and have a philosophy that looks more to total use of drugs and the patient's personality and life style; these have been more ready to condemn marijuana use, and to forbid it among their patients.

It is difficult in treatment programs to forbid behavior where transgressions cannot be monitored with some regularity and where detection of abuse is more or less fortuitous. Forbidden behavior, if constantly practiced, tends to generalize and creates a climate of disrespect for the rules of the organization as well as creating a climate of unfairness for the occasional individual who gets caught and who can rightfully say that he is being scapegoated (i.e. that many other people are doing the forbidden behavior).

The presence of a reliable, inexpensive and easily performed test for marijuana could change this picture and require programs to rethink their attitudes toward such behavior. I predict that such a change would be in the direction of reinforcing present tendencies. Therapeutic communities will find the technique a useful tool to enforce the prohibition. Methadone programs are more likely not to use the technique or to find it useful only in certain specific circumstances (e.g. where marijuana use would be seen as very deleterious, such as clients with a history of schizophrenia, or paranoia).

Outpatient adolescent programs will probably have the most problems with the new technique. Current surveys of use indicate that most of their clients will use marijuana at least occasionally and a substantial number on a regular basis. The new test will make it possible for programs to detect and focus on such use, even when it may be more important to look at other aspects of the adolescents' lives and relationships. Parents and legal officials may put pressure on programs to enforce total abstinence from marijuana in spite of the real possibility that such demands will be counterproductive and lead to program estrangement.

One difficulty involved with using the EMIT assay has to do with the duration of THC in the urine. As the summary report notes, "with the EMIT Cannabinoid Assay it is not possible to distinguish between very recent use (within 24 hours) and recent use (up to 10 days)." This persistence will permit patients to use for a number of days after being initially detected without the program being certain whether use has occurred before or after the infraction. This uncertainty can lead to unproductive client-staff arguments which detract from and deflect attention from more crucial therapeutic issues.

There is the question in drug treatment programs of having to deal with relative dangers, competing priorities and treatment issues, and of the occasional to moderate use of a substance widely used and widely tolerated by the larger community with whom the patients are in contact. Programs will have to decide whether any use equals abuse or whether the laboratory findings will be primarily confirmatory of an abuse situation defined behaviorally.

URINE TESTING FOR MARIJUANA USE: IMPLICATIONS IN CORRECTIONS

Hugh Alcott,
Special Narcotics Section,
California Department of Corrections

Institutional Application

The control of drug use and drug trafficking has long been a problem in the management of correctional institutions. The use of drugs can lead to many problems such as trafficking by inmate groups who use the money to finance their other gang activities. Now that an accurate, inexpensive on-site method exists to test inmate urines for marijuana as well as most other drugs, the question of application arises. Once an institution decides to implement marijuana testing the first thing is to decide what will be done with the test results. A program of reasonable sanctions must be established and agreed on by staff and then fairly and uniformly applied. A system of random urine testing must be established that is consistently followed and allows for additional testing for cause.

The following is an operational procedure laid out by the California Department of Corrections for urine testing in our institutions:

- *General Procedure:* Two random urine specimens are taken per day per dorm and tested for opiates and THC, and occasionally tested fully. Up to 50 specimens may be taken per day for "good cause." These samples will be tested for one specific substance.
- *Civil Addicts:* For a first positive drug use result the following actions will be taken: (1) refer to district attorney for prosecution; (2) issue notice; (3) refer to unit and institution classification review committees for review and for certification to the Narcotic Addict Evaluation Authority. For a second positive drug use result: (1) refer to district attorney; (2) issue notice; (3) refer to classification review committee and to exclusion review committee for possible decision to exclude from program.
- *Felons:* For a first positive drug use result: (1) refer to district attorney for prosecution; (2) issue serious notice; (3) consider loss of 10 days credit; and (4) refer for program review. For a second posi-

tive drug use result: (1) refer to district attorney; (2) issue serious notice; (3) consider loss of 15 days credit; and (4) refer to committee for possible transfer to another institution.

When we first started using the marijuana test, the incidence of positive tests was as high as 30% of any given group of urines. Six weeks following the start of the routine marijuana testing with administrative sanctions applied, the positive level dropped to less than 8%.

The use of the marijuana test and the application of reasonable sanctions has given our institution a control tool that is working. We have tested more than 5,000 inmate urines for cannabis metabolites and feel that our testing protocol is very productive as a control tool.

Parole Applications

In California, those parolees whose past record indicates a history of drug abuse are required, as a condition of parole, to participate in urine testing. In the past four and one-half years, more than 200,000 urine drug tests have been done by our on-site EMIT labs. While more than 3,000 parolee urines have been tested for marijuana resulting in a positive rate of about 40%, no formal sanctions have yet been established but are being reviewed at this time.

The basic question is: How important is marijuana use among a parole population and what sanctions, if any, are indicated? We ran a survey to see if there was any relationship between the use of marijuana and the use of other drugs, among a parole population of pre-identified drug abusers. Over a period of 30 days, we tested 396 urines (225 parolees) for marijuana, opiates and PCP. Fifty-seven persons tested negative for all drugs; 78 persons tested positive for cannabinoids only; and 90 persons tested positive for cannabis and other drugs.

Summary

When any branch of the criminal justice system, charged with the treatment and control of drug users/abusers, uses the marijuana test as a tool, they must be ready to deal with test results; they must follow a strict protocol, and have reasonable sanctions, consistently and fairly applied.

Discussion and Responses to Questions

Regarding the large-scale testing of the EMIT Cannabinoid Assay in the California prison system, Mr. Alcott added the following remarks. In California, urine testing among pre-identified drug users leaving prison is a legal condition of parole; there are no personal privacy prohibitions. Because drugs are not permitted in prisons, observed urines are permissable, which eliminates to the extent possible such practices as switching urines, adulterating urines, etc. Thus, the prison system seemed ideal for a large-scale test of the EMIT Cannabinoid Assay. Between October, 1979 and October, 1980 over 10,000 EMIT assays were conducted, with 40% showing positive. Of these, 25% were prisoners, 75% were parolees. Because of the cost of GC/MS screening ($50.00 per urine), positives were not validated. However, when the 4,000 prisoners and parolees were confronted with their positive scores, only three denied using marijuana.

When the testing for marijuana started, there was a great deal of concern expressed by both staff and inmates as to the accuracy of the test and the technology itself. Briefing meetings were held with the Inmate Advisory Council. The pre-identified drug-user inmate population was given three weeks notice. All were taken through the laboratory where both the technology and its operation were explained and demonstrated. The intent was to remove any mystery and show the test for what it is: an accurate, well-applied testing method.

Although California was the first to use EMIT for a broad-based evaluation, criminal justice systems in Oregon, Missouri and Alaska are now applying it. California regards the assay as a control tool which is used more for preventive purposes than for punitive purposes. Punishment has to be an available alternative (classifications can be changed, visiting privileges taken away, time before seeing the parole board extended, or inmates can be transferred), but other modalities should be tried first. California regards EMIT as a measuring tool, which measures progress as well as recidivism.

Question: Did the test of 10,000 urines show any findings about passive ingestion of marijuana?

Response: The department conducted a non-controlled, non-scientific test of the "passive ingestion" defense, and, after enclosing smokers and non-smokers in a car for several hours, found that none of the non-smokers had positive indications.

Question: Are there any problems with the EMIT Cannabinoid Assay which others should be aware of?

Response: Regarding problems with the EMIT assay, it behooves systems to scrutinize closely how operators are trained, and to provide controls and follow-up procedures for monitoring operators.

MARIJUANA TESTING – IMPLICATIONS FOR HIGHWAY SAFETY

The two papers presented on this subject showed a basic disagreement on measurements of marijuana-related driving impairment, a disagreement of degree and emphasis, based in part on test objectives and procedures. However, the two prominent researchers with extensive experience in drug/driving research, Dr. Arthur J. McBay and Dr. Herbert Moskowitz, agreed that urine testing, by itself, would not be sufficient to support a deterrence program, principally because urinalysis will not produce measures of intoxication. Dr. McBay said the literature on the effects of marijuana on driving indicates that the effects are subtle and variable with the majority of subjects showing some evidence of deterioration of performance and other subjects showing improvement or no change in performance. Dr. Moskowitz noted that "in studies which have multiple dose levels, the effects are clearly dose related, with greater amounts of marijuana producing a greater degree of impairment."

MARIJUANA AND DRIVING

Herbert Moskowitz, Ph.D.
Professor of Psychology
California State University at Los Angeles
and University of California

The three major road vehicle studies (Hanstein et al, Klonoff et al, and Atwood) have all demonstrated that marijuana produces impairment in car control. Typically these effects only appear clearly at doses of roughly 100 micrograms delta-9-THC per kg body weight.* However, these studies utilized short duration runs in relatively restricted environments without the demands for visual search that typify actual driving.

Results from driving simulator studies have suggested a greater magnitude of impairment. Raphaelsen found that 12 mg of THC produced substantial increases in the latency of brake and accelerator responses to the appearance of traffic signals. Moskowitz et al found dose-related increases in reaction time to light signals and in incorrect responses, begin-

*Dosage levels in physiological studies are usually reported as amount of drug administered per kg of body weight. One hundred micrograms delta-9-THC per kg body weight corresponds to 7 mg given to a 70 kg (154 lb) subject.

ning at 50 micrograms THC per kg, but only a small effect on tracking.

In a complex closed-loop computer-controlled driving simulator which provides a more accurate representation of the tracking demand of actual driving over a wide range of roads (conducted by Moskowitz and colleagues), 15 subjects drove 45 minutes under 0, 100 or 200 micrograms THC per kg. Marijuana produced increasing variability in lateral lane position while proceeding through curves and while being buffeted by winds. Both the frequency and duration of time spent by subjects outside the lane increased in a dose-related fashion. Subjects found it difficult to maintain the requested constant speed in curves. The ability to maintain a constant distance headway while following a car also declined. An emergency situation involving the sudden appearance of a roadway obstacle produced two crashes during the placebo condition but seven and 14 crashes for the low and high marijuana doses, respectively.

MARIJUANA AND HIGHWAY SAFETY

by Arthur J. McBay, Ph.D.
Professor of Pathology and Pharmacy, University of North Carolina, and Chief Toxicologist, Office of the Chief Medical Examiner, Chapel Hill, North Carolina

The literature does not reveal that marijuana is a factor in unsafe operation of a motor vehicle. Sparse as the reports may be, they tend to show that if there are drivers who are unsafe because of marijuana, that their numbers are small and that most are also influenced by alcohol.

- Crancer, 1969: The subjects under the influence of alcohol made significantly more simulator errors than under control conditions. The only simulator error made by marijuana smokers was an increase in speedometer errors. No increase in impairment was noted because of inexperienced marijuana users or when marijuana dosage was increased. About half of the subjects showed improvement in error scores following marijuana smoking.
- Dott, 1972: It appears (in a test of risk acceptance using a simulated passing task) that the subject under the influence of marijuana was less likely to accept the increased risk of attempting to make hazardous passes. Marijuana did not significantly affect the emergency decision reaction time or the

lateral control of the vehicle. A similar study using alcohol revealed a very significant deterioration of performance and risk acceptance.

- Klonoff, 1974: At the highest dosage of marijuana used, driving performance significantly declined in 63% of the drivers, 21% showed no change, and 16% significantly improved.
- Teale, 1977: In an examination of 66 bloods obtained from fatally injured drivers, THC was found in 3 of the bloods.
- Moskowitz, 1976: (A driving simulator was used.) The drug did not create significant deviations from the norm in car control and tracking, nor was an increase in reaction time observed as the dose was increased. There was an increase in reaction time in response to signal lights.
- Cimbura, 1980: THC was found in the bloods of 14 (3.5%) of 401 fatally injured drivers, but 7 of the 14 had more than 0.09% alcohol in their blood. The bloods of 2 of the drivers contained 5 ng/ml of THC, the rest had less than 3 ng/ml.

The blood specimens of 169 operators killed in single vehicle accidents in North Carolina were examined for alcohol, marijuana and other drugs. More than 0.09% alcohol was found in 67% of the bloods and some alcohol was found in 12% more. THC was found in the bloods of 10 drivers (6%), but 8 of these contained more than 0.08% alcohol.

Documentation of a significant adverse effect of marijuana smoking on highway safety has not been found. Studies are needed which relate the concentration of THC in the blood to effects. The presence of cannabinoids in the breath or saliva may indicate recent smoking, but probably does not relate to psychological effects. After a single exposure to marijuana, cannabinoids will persist in the urine for a day or two to a week or more. Analytical results must be based on valid, well-controlled, confirmed tests performed by competent analysts.

The present state of knowledge indicates that marijuana smoking may cause some subtle deterioration of driving performance in the majority of drivers, but a large minority will show no change or impairment. Preliminary and limited reports indicate that the number of drivers found who could have been adversely affected by marijuana is very small compared to the number of those adversely affected by alcohol and most of them are also under the influence of alcohol.

Thus, in the driving simulator, significant impairments were found in car control. However, under marijuana, subjects appeared more conservative. When requested to pass cars, they would only attempt the task with a greater than normal distance to the approaching vehicle.

Another major aspect of driving is perception, the ability to detect and recognize potential dangers such as other vehicles, traffic signals or pedestrians. In general, while simple visual functions show only minor effects under marijuana, signal recognition and vigilance show considerable impairment.

In a recently completed study two tracking tasks were examined, a compensatory tracking task and a critical tracking task (which is an unstable and increasingly difficult task). While the simpler compensatory task was impaired at the high dose for a period of up to three hours, the more sensitive critical tracking task showed impairment at all dose levels. Morever, at the higher dose level, the impairment remained significant for almost 10 hours.

Several studies examined joint alcohol-marijuana administration. In all cases, the effects clearly have been at least additive, with marijuana increasing the alcohol-induced impairments.

What can be done to suppress marijuana use and driving? The most relevant suggestions come from the extensive research on alcohol and driving where the prime method of suppression is through deterrence by threat of arrest and punishment. However, this requires bringing a driver into court and demonstrating his blood alcohol concentration was sufficient to produce significant impairment. This demonstration rests on an extensive research literature relating the degree of driving impairment and accident probability to blood alcohol levels. The literature demonstrates that this relationship holds substantially true regardless of when the alcohol was consumed.

Given the widespread prevalence of the alcohol model, it would appear likely that successful legal prosecution upon which deterrence depends requires a THC blood level and a demonstration that that level is meaningfully related over the time of THC's appearance in the blood to the degree of driving impairment. No such evidence is currently available.

While the studies mentioned above have shown that driving impairment is correlated with the dose administered, these studies mainly tested behavior in the first hour or so after administration. It is not clear if the correlation of dose administered to degree of impairment will continue to hold as the drug is recirculated through the body and the relative distribution of metabolites changes.

Given that these problems remain even before an

accurate test of blood THC levels could be utilized, what can be said for a cannabinoid urine test that is essentially uncorrelated with blood levels?

Such a urine test might be a simple precursor screen to a subsequent demand for a blood test, or a research tool to determine the number of drivers who are marijuana users, but, in and of itself, it would not appear to support a deterrence program to suppress driving while under the influence of marijuana.

JUVENILE MARIJUANA USE

It is useful to consider the following three papers within a common framework. While their subject areas range from schools to pediatrics to general prevention, each of the three addresses the issue of broadly based testing of school-age youth.

REMARKS ON PREVENTION

William L. Barton
President, National Federation of Parents for Drug Free Youth

Today's parents are relatively ignorant and naive on the subject of drugs. Conversely, today's teenager lives in a world permeated by drugs and the typical teenager possesses a great deal of information about drugs. Unfortunately, much of that information is grossly inaccurate. Since the use of drugs by children is generally considered unacceptable behavior and is illegal, young persons using drugs will attempt to hide these activities from any authoritative entity, and, in the absence of positive proof, will lie to cover up their use of drugs.

It is extremely difficult, if not impossible, for even trained experts to detect drug usage in its early stages simply by observation. The net result is that millions of young Americans are using drugs for extended periods without the knowledge of their parents, millions of kids whose drug usage is not detected until it has become a serious problem.

In order for a parent to intervene "early" in a child's drug usage, that parent must first become aware of the drug usage. We, the National Federation of Parents, are convinced that tools such as the EMIT urine test can play a major role in early detection.

Several things must happen, however, for this type of test to approach its full potential. First, the test must become a routine part of all physical examinations for children in grades 6 (even lower in certain areas) through 12; second, the parents of children whose test results are positive must be informed of the results.

Such a program would vastly increase the instances of early detection – early intervention with potentially thousands of young Americans being spared the horrors of serious drug problems.

We would also expect simple detection tests, such as EMIT, to become a deterrent to drug use. It seems reasonable that if simple detection tests were routinely employed, a significant percentage of our youth who are currently saying "yes" to drugs would instead say "no."

URINE SCREEN FOR CANNABINOIDS – A PEDIATRIC VIEW

Donald I. Macdonald, M.D.
Clinical Associate Professor of Pediatrics
University of South Florida

Urine testing for marijuana use should be employed in routine clinical examination of sick children, for annual checkups and for clinical follow-up.

An adolescent who is brought to the pediatrician with symptoms of fatigue should be suspected of using drugs especially if he has suggestive behavior and appearance. Testing for cannabinoids could be at least as important in establishing a diagnosis and outlining treatment as are the tests commonly used to detect anemia, mononucleosis, or hepatitis. Likewise the child brought in with chronic cough, sore throat, or red eyes should be screened for marijuana use as readily as he is tested for other possibilities.

Children are often great con artists and it is frequently difficult to know when they are using pot and when they are not. For those children known to have been involved who are undergoing behavior modification either at home or in a more formal setting, this test may have real value.

Treatment programs have less than 100% success rate and are at best expensive and time consuming. A better answer has to lie in prevention or detection and treatment in early stages of involvement. Parental awareness and adolescent denial can both be addressed by a reliable screening examination.

At issue are children's rights, protection of children, parental rights and responsibilities, confidentiality of information, and communicability of disease. Adolescent drug use/abuse is an epidemic and contagious disease of major proportions. Children's rights are being violated by a massive commercial push to involve them in drugs and they must be protected. Parents need the tools to protect their children. There is little need to test children who are admitted marijuana smokers and there is no break in confidentiality in revealing to parents information about illegal activity about which the child has lied. Precedent does exist for the use of mandatory detection procedures to assist in control of dangerous disease.

False positives may be checked by another method but this is not always practical. Of more concern are false negatives which will allow a child more strongly to deny involvement and may give the parents a false sense of security. This writer has reason to feel from his own practice that there may be false negative diagnoses in the adolescent age group. These few cases may reflect erroneous clinical impression, improper handling and storing of urine samples in the office, or laboratory error. They may also be related to altered metabolism or relative unsaturation of alternate binding sites in patients.

If the concern related here can be resolved and urine testing for cannabinoids does prove to be reliable and inexpensive, the pediatrician will have a great new weapon in his child care armamentarium.

IMPLICATIONS OF URINE TESTING FOR MARIJUANA IN A SCHOOL SETTING

Richard A. Hawley, Ph.D.
Dean of Students, The University School
Cleveland, Ohio

The finding (according to NIDA's 1979 study, *Drugs and the Nation's High School Students*) that substantial numbers of the nation's young people between ages 11 and 18 are partaking of millions, and possibly billions, of dollars worth of an illicit drug may in itself constitute an important social and political problem. A more important concern stems from the toxicity of marijuana's principal psychoactive chemical, delta-9-THC.

It is not disputed that THC acts on various neural processes to produce an altered feeling state, or "high." Various conceptual schemes are being formulated to link laboratory research showing neural damage with clinical observations of long-term personality alterations such as the "amotivational syndrome," depression, vagueness, and hyper-irritability.

Over the past 15 years, some clinical psychologists, educators and other, less specialized observers, with or without a sound neurological basis, have been associating youthful marijuana use with diminishing school performance and various personality disorders. School personnel have not been able, nor will they be able in the future, to ignore the phenomenon of widespread use of psychoactive drugs in the schools. It is unavoidably true that marijuana use causes school problems which are both immediate and long-range, and derive both from the drug's immediate psychoactive properties and from the more remote effects of long-term storage in the cells of the nervous system.

Stoned students are passive, inattentive, and otherwise inappropriate in a structured learning setting. More than just the interests of stoned students are at stake. The pot user's lack of attentiveness and disengagement contribute to a classroom atmosphere in which engagement of other class members is less likely. Teachers are confronted with what they perceive to be uninterested, hostile or inadequate pupils and become frustrated sooner when student responses are not forthcoming. It is perhaps no accident that the phenomenon of "teacher burnout" has followed directly on the heels of widespread marijuana use by school-aged children. Moreover, once-standard curricula cannot be mastered by drug-altered students and may be abandoned in favor of less-challenging curricula. Again, it may be no accident that the cultural changes that followed in the wake of widespread drug use by students required less demonstrated competence as a condition of course credit, diplomas, and other school credentials. Accompanying these changes has been steadily declining competence as measured by national test scores and as reported by concerned educators at the junior high school, high school, and undergraduate levels.

Three kinds of learning losses result from student cannabis use, (1) the loss of course content and of new skills due to the user's being high during instruction; (2) the long-term slowing of arousal, the flattening of outward affect, and the impairment of memory and analytical abilities that come with chronic use; and (3) retardation of the emotional development necessary to attain adulthood.

The chronic marijuana user is accruing THC faster than it is being metabolized and eliminated from the body. Thus, after several months, the user is "fat-saturated" with cannabinoids and is never free of the drug's effects, including the neurological ones that bear most on learning. Formerly adequate students who use marijuana regularly become, often in a few months, passive, irritable, and delinquent. These behavioral changes become classroom and disciplinary concerns.

Because the marijuana problem is inevitably a school problem, the urine test for recent cannabis consumption may have some useful applications in that setting. There is not yet a shared pool of reliable information about marijuana's effects or a shared professional conviction that marijuana poses a danger to health and learning. A consensus among educators may be constructed in the foreseeable future. In the meantime, it is often difficult for school personnel to talk frankly with students whose marijuana use is suspected or apparent. Such students often fear disciplinary reprisals if they admit marijuana involvement.

Counselors and teachers who would like to demonstrate the relationship between a student's marijuana use and specific problem behaviors would be aided considerably by having their observations confirmed (or not) by a urine test.

The school itself, however, seems an inappropriate place in which to administer such a test.

A workable model of the process in which the school and the student might now benefit from the urine testing might be as follows:

- A teacher or counselor identifies a student problem he either knows or suspects to be marijuana-related.
- The teacher/counselor shares the concern with the student in a non-disciplinary setting.
- The teacher/counselor contacts the family of the student to discuss the problem and proposes that the parents have the child urine-tested for recent marijuana use by a physician (perhaps as part of a general physical examination).
- If/when the testing results are positive, then counselor, family and student can further explore the relationship between marijuana use and the problem identified. Moratoriums on use and other family-student policies can be implemented as the teacher/counselor monitors changes in school performance.

For such a process to work, a school-parent-physician partnership would have to be formed which takes considerable time, commitment, and a willingness on the part of all three to consider marijuana use as a causal factor in the student's problem.

Alternatively, if pediatricians and other physicians attending school-aged youth would routinely urine-test school-aged children for cannabis metabolites in the course of physical examinations, then positive results, when correlated by parents with school and behavior problems, might be countered with parental sanctions.

It may be instructive to note that for students of my

acquaintance who have been referred to neurologists for a brain wave scan due to a concern about marijuana use, the experience of being tested for neural damage helped many of them to stop using the drug.

Becoming aware that a complex chemical compound enters several of the internal organs and proceeds to affect each before slowly metabolizing is often an important step in a young person's looking critically at what has been for him a strictly sensual and social experience.

I suggest a school-family-physician partnership on marijuana problems because, given the public's spotty awareness of the biomedical effects of cannabis, a more compulsory application of urine testing might raise thorny civil liberties issues, which would actually impede the formation of any future social consensus that marijuana is a hazard to the health and education of the young.

When such a consensus is established, then the uses of urine testing might be very different. For example, once it is widely acknowledged that marijuana users are unable to contribute to classroom work and to school life in general, it might, depending on a community's commitment to educational quality, be conceivable that a negative test result be required as a condition of any student's enrollment in school. It is easy to imagine such a policy being adopted at least with respect to chronic violators of a school's established marijuana rules.

It cannot be over-emphasized that any school policy which would recommend or require such tests rests on the strength of its conviction that marijuana use significantly impairs learning and the school process in general.

Discussion and Responses to Questions on Juvenile Marijuana Use

Regarding the legal considerations in the testing of minors, Nancy Wynstra commented that various uses of the urine test would have to be evaluated legally on a case-by-case, state-by-state basis. One state's courts might sanction a specific use, whereas the courts in another state might abridge or curtail that use. Testing a youngster in a doctor's office at the parent's request is probably acceptable. However, many states have laws which permit juveniles to restrict parental access to information concerning their involvement in drug treatment programs. Thus, in some states, physicians might be prohibitied from sharing the drug test information with a parent unless the minor child consents.

Dr. Macdonald offered the following pediatric pointers for using the EMIT Assay. Most kids are not "up" on methods of adulterating or switching urine samples. Consequently, the pediatrician need not feel that the only valid urine test comes from an observed urine. Nevertheless, precautions should be taken. Soap, half-filled coffee cups and other tempting "adulterators" should be removed from the bathroom where the urine specimen is delivered. If the physician suspects that the urine has been altered, ask for another sample immediately. If the patient says he can't, offer water or fruit juice, and ask him to wait. A series of objections or stalls should be noted, as should pale urines, which can be pre-adulterated if the patient drinks a good deal of liquid beforehand.

Question: Are pediatricians obligated to ask permission before giving the test?

Response: Wynstra: Physicians are not obligated to ask permission before giving the urine test, any more than they are obligated to ask permission before giving any number of other tests that they deem necessary. However, if the parent or child asks whether the test is to be given, the physician is obligated to explain why.

Question: What is the probability of formulating an approval protocol for physicians wishing to contribute to a controlled study along these lines?

Response: Dr. Macdonald: NIDA has agreed to serve as a focal point (through Dr. Ingrid Lantner) in receiving clinical reports from family physicians, parents and teachers on changes in health and development seen in chronic marijuana-smoking youngsters. The use of marijuana and other drugs during early adolescence, the period of most rapid physical and psychological development, is of particular concern. This material will aid in evaluating the consequences of marijuana use among pubertal and older youngsters; it will also be an important indicator of what additional, more structured research needs to be undertaken.

Question: Have any controlled studies been conducted on chronic adolescent male pot smokers to substantiate research findings which have shown lowered testosterone levels among adult male chronic smokers?

Response: Dr. Macdonald: Our clinical research program is planning to conduct a test of testosterone levels in adolescents with positive results of cannabis indicated by urinalysis.

Question: Would it be helpful for physicians, pediatricians and obstetricians immediately to run an EMIT urine test on mothers who produce low weight babies to see whether there might be any correlation between this and pregnant pot smoking women?

Response: Dr. Macdonald: I would strongly support anything we can do to shed further light on the problems of low-weight babies or congenital defects and their possible relation to marijuana. A further point regarding low-weight babies is this: they are particularly a problem in the case of teen-aged mothers because these young girls are not physiologically mature, and we know that drug-using adolescents are more socially active and less careful of the consequences. I've been aware of how many mothers have given up drinking during pregnancy. If those who smoke marijuana realized the hazards to their baby, they'd be more apt to give that up too – except perhaps in the case of teenagers who have less will power and self-control. It's important that controlled studies be done in this area. In the meantime, the more education of the mother-to-be, the better, so far as possible negative consequences of marijuana smoking during pregnancy are concerned.

Question: In counselling in the schools, how effective is information on the health hazards of marijuana? Can information alone cause a student to give up pot smoking?

Response: Dr. Hawley: Information on the health hazards of marijuana can induce a student to give up smoking, particularly if the user isn't too involved with the drug. Most youngsters are interested in their own health – especially if you don't come on from the disciplinary standpoint first.

IMPLICATIONS FOR MARIJUANA TESTING IN THE WORKPLACE AND THE MILITARY

A representative of Ford Motor Company's employee health services counseling program, and the chief surgeon of a railway system were adamant in expressing industry opinion that drug usage or trafficking cannot be tolerated in the workplace. A spokesman for the military added that "cannabis is our next biggest problem (after alcohol) due primarily to prevalence of use." Following are three papers on these topics.

URINE TESTING FOR MARIJUANA: IMPLICATIONS FOR THE WORKPLACE

James L. Francek, MSW, ACSW
Corporate Coordinator, Employee Health Services Counseling, Ford Motor Company

An employer should expect a full day's work for a full day's wage. When an employee falls below standard levels of performance or attendance, he or she can be held accountable for that failure. A consistent system of accountability joined with a consistent offer of quality medical help often results in dramatic positive change of the impaired individual. Companies cannot condone illegal activities within their boundaries. The observed sale or use of marijuana is illegal. In most companies, it results in termination. This action has been further backed up through various arbitration actions. The observed impairment of an employee under the influence of alcohol or drugs presents a serious safety problem within the workplace. Federal and state safety legislation charge the employer with the maintenance of a safe workplace. The removal of persons who are "unsafe in the workplace" establishes serious legal and ethical mandates. Persons found to be unsafe because of their misuse of alcohol or drugs may be subject to normal disiplinary procedures. Regular (daily) users will eventually become serious safety problems.

Before urine testing for marijuana becomes commonplace in the workplace, a number of crucial program considerations must be reviewed:

- *Policy.* The leaders must develop an overall policy. The sensitive question of observed use or sale must be differentiated from the observed impairment of an individual.
- *Procedures.* Once a policy has been arrived at, procedures for referral for testing must be clearly communicated to everyone.
- *Role Delineation.* The various roles of referral persons must be appropriately spelled out. Non-clinical personnel should not be charged with clinical procedures.
- *Problem Resolution.* Once impaired individuals are identified, an appropriate method of resolution should be placed before them.

All of the program considerations above are dependent on the validity, specificity and reliability of the testing procedure.

The following represents a list of questions confronting business leaders which should be answered in developing appropriate policy:

- What are the assumptions and consequences of refusing a urine test?
- Will this test be used for clinical clarification or a witch hunt?
- Are there any clinical tests that can separate the synergistic effects of multiple drug use? (alcohol, marijuana, valium, etc.).
- At what levels of marijuana use can we assume in-

toxication and unsafeness?

- At what stage of marijuana use is treatment needed? What types of treatment are available?
- When should the test be administered? By whom? Who gets the report?
- What are the confidentiality considerations of such a test?
- What role does a person's physical tolerance to the drug have in relationship to an established standard of impairment?
- Will the existence of the test and referral procedures in the workplace overcome the fear that supervisors have of the drug user?
- How long can employers and unions tolerate the increased prevalence of marijuana and still maintain quality and consistency?
- What are the legal considerations of releasing an impaired individual to drive himself or herself home?

REMARKS

Max D. Rogers, M.D.
Chief Surgeon
Southern Railway System

Dr. Rogers explained the railroads' "Rule G" which, for 150 years, has stipulated that any person caught on duty under the influence of alcohol could be summarily dismissed without recourse. Dr. Rogers noted that Rule G has been broadened to include other substances that "do not mix with a business involving heavy equipment, speed and momentum." The following is an abstract of Dr. Rogers' paper.

With the advent of urine screen tests, we were able to determine readily whether or not a person was under the influence of various drugs. But we were increasingly aware that some employees were using a substance for which we could not test, namely marijuana. There was no evidence to sustain a charge under Rule G. With no way to test, we had no statistics on the extent of marijuana use by our people. Now that we do have a urine screen test for marijuana, we have a tool not only to define the problem but also to deal with it.

About 3,000 of our front-line supervisors were advised that if they had reason to suspect that one of our people was using marijuana, that person should be taken to a company physician and a urine screen requested.

Actually, we have had very few of these tests for marijuana run since then. My hunch is that the knowledge that we can now test for marijuana has been and will be a strong deterrent to our employees using it on duty.

Our police department and our legal staff are working together to develop procedures for dealing with marijuana possession by our employees who are on duty but are staying in company dormitories during layover or turnaround periods. They would like to see possession of marijuana be just as strong a cause for dismissal as the use of it.

It is literally impossible to calculate how many lives have been saved by Rule G, how much suffering and damage avoided. When hard drugs were added to the list of Rule G prohibitions, we found a decrease in the use of cocaine, heroin, morphine, demerol and others. My firm belief is that with marijuana on the prohibited list, and our people aware that we can test for it, we will also see a decline in the use of this drug.

In the railroad industry, we feel that the use of any intoxicant, narcotic or hallucinatory substance by men and women on duty is simply unacceptable. The risks are too great, for all of us.

REMARKS

William C. Louisell, Brig. Gen., U.S. Army (Ret.)
Deputy Assistant to Secretary of Defense
for Drug and Alcohol Abuse Prevention

General Louisell presented background information on the nature of the alcohol and drug problem in the military, outlined the focus of the Department of Defense policy toward alcohol and drug abuse among military personnel, and discussed how urine testing fits into overall DoD policy and programs.

Cannabis is our next biggest problem (after alcohol) due primarily to prevalence of use. The following data support this contention.

- 26% of tested military personnel used cannabis in the last 30 days, including 37% of the younger enlisted personnel.
- 19% have used cannabis weekly or more often, including 31% of the younger enlisted personnel.
- 17% are high more than one day at a time.
- 19% have been high while working at least once.
- 21% have reported some work impairment.

The Pentagon's primary goal is to be free of the adverse effects of alcohol and drug abuse (the Department spends more than $95 million a year on its prevention, treatment and rehabilitiation program). The current marijuana urine testing methodology provides "a reliable means of identifying persons who have not used cannabis within the last two weeks – this in itself is helpful for screening people for critical jobs – and a means of tentatively identifying those who have." The results should be confirmed by alternative methods such as gas chromatography/mass spectrometry.

If the urine testing systems are approved, the military would use them "in situations in which suspicion of drug abuse arises – AWOLs, failure to obey lawful orders; deterioration, abnormal or bizarre behavior; assault; safety violations; apprehensions or investigations for drug offenses, etc." Again, positive results would have to be confirmed by laboratories, and the military would probably not use the urine testing systems for mass screening or "sweep" testing.

The military needs a means of identifying persons who are under the influence of cannabis, but current technology cannot meet this need because there is no correlation between urine metabolites and level of impairment, and the methods cannot distinguish between very recent use and use of up to 10 days before testing.

Similarly, the military needs a means of identifying persons who are heavy users of cannabis, under the presumption that this heavy use may cause unreliability, a need that the urine testing methodology also does not meet.

The Department of Defense is currently testing three portable urine testing kits with results due sometime in 1981.

Discussion and Responses to Questions on the Implications of Marijuana Testing in the Workplace and the Military

Regarding the legal considerations for testing in the workplace, Nancy Wynstra commented that the test could probably be used legally in certain employment settings, so long as the decision to administer the test was triggered by a concrete event, e.g., the employee's apparent intoxication, or the employee being found using a substance reasonably believed to be marijuana. The test would probably withstand legal scrutiny if it could be demonstrated that any marijuana use significantly compromised the employee's ability to perform duties. Law enforcement officers, persons involved in national security, or employees whose jobs have serious safety implications would be examples. Still, testing programs would have to be carefully structured to withstand legal challenges.

Question: Dr. Rogers, how often is Rule G applied by your outfit in a year? Gen. Louisell, how many military personnel were discharged last year or sent to treatment?

Response: Dr. Rogers: The Southern discharges about five employees a year. "The solution is the employees' assistance programs. . . . We've been working very carefully and closely with the unions in our drug and alcohol programs, and we've promised the union representatives that, if a person is discharged under Rule G, and if he accepts appropriate treatment and recovers, he may apply for reinstatement. We have alcoholics back on duty who were discharged under Rule G."

Response: Gen. Louisell: Some 25,000 military members were detected by various means in 1980, referred to treatment and rehabilitation and returned to service. There were 74 discharges.

Question: How about offering treatment as an alternative to discharge?

Response: Dr. Rogers: Offering treatment as an alternative to discharge is a plausible answer, but Rule G has worked well since 1840. "You're out; you go take the treatment; but come back. We feel this is a great deterrent to their usage on duty. It's very rare that we fire an employee on the first case; generally, it's a suspension."

Question: What is the potential for random urine testing in industry?

Response: Mr. Francek: "It could prove useful since we seem to have a dual value system. Alcohol use is far more readily picked up. The drug addict tends to be overlooked or forgotten because there haven't been adequate tools to work with; also because there is a lot of stigma in working with them due to fear of violence. These folks are therefore often allowed to progress to their late stages. If, however, the drug user were faced early on with the facts and consequences of his drug use, chances are he would accept help earlier, and get better earlier."

Question: What are the legal considerations of pre-employment pot test screening? Also, could Rule G be applied to such critical areas as nuclear plants? What about daily screening in highly sensitive areas?

Response: Nancy Wynstra: "Unless it was some highly technical, super-critical area – critical to our entire civilization, I don't think daily testing would stand up. For pre-employment screening, you'd have to have a rationale about why it is important to know whether they use this drug. If you could show, for example, that employees who had tested positive for marijuana use had a five-fold accident increase over those who tested negative, this would probably justify using the cannabinoid test as a criterion for exclusion from employment. However, if you're talking about increased absenteeism of clerks from a department store, I doubt that would be regarded as sufficiently critical socially to warrant that kind of intrusion in personal rights."

Booklets Available From the American Council for Drug Education

Blasinsky, M. and Russell, G. K. (Eds.) *Urine Testing for Marijuana Use: Implications for a Variety of Settings.* American Council on Marijuana, New York; $2.50.

Cohen, S. *Cocaine Today.* American Council on Marijuana, New York; $2.50.

Cohen, S. and Andrysiak, T. *Therapeutic Potential of Marijuana's Components.* American Council on Marijuana, New York; $2.50.

Cohen, S. and Lessin, P. J. *Marijuana and Alcohol.* American Council on Marijuana, New York; $2.50.

de Silva, R. and DuPont, R. L. (Eds.) *Treating the Marijuana-Dependent Person.* American Council on Marijuana, New York; $2.95.

Heath, R. G. *Marijuana and the Brain.* American Council on Marijuana, New York; $1.50.

Lantner, I. and Barth, R. *A Pediatrician's View of Marijuana,* American Council on Marijuana, New York; $2.50.

Marijuana: *The National Impact on Education.* American Council on Marijuana, New York; $2.95.

Moskowitz, H. and Petersen, R. *Marijuana and Driving.* American Council on Marijuana, New York; $2.50.

Petersen, R., Cohen, S., Jeri, F. R., Smith, D., and Dogoloff, L. *Cocaine: A Second Look.* American Council on Marijuana, New York; $2.50.

Russell, G. K. *Marijuana Today: A Compilation of Medical Findings for the Layman.* The Myrin Institute, New York; $3.00.

Smith, C. G. and Asch, R. H. *Marijuana and Reproduction.* American Council on Marijuana, New York; $2.50.

Tashkin, D. P. and Cohen, S. *Marijuana Smoking and Its Effects on the Lungs.* American Council on Marijuana, New York; $2.50.

Turner, C. E. *The Marijuana Controversy: Definition, Research Perspective and Therapeutic Claims.* American Council on Marijuana, New York; $1.99.

Free catalog on additional materials and films available upon written request.